The New
Self Help Series
BAD BREATH

The New Self Help Series
BAD BREATH

LEON CHAITOW
N.D., D.O.

Thorsons
An Imprint of HarperCollinsPublishers

Thorsons
An Imprint of HarperCollins*Publishers*
77–85 Fulham Palace Road,
Hammersmith, London W6 8JB

Published by Thorsons 1994
10 9 8 7 6 5 4 3 2 1

© Leon Chaitow 1994

Leon Chaitow asserts the moral right to
be identified as the author of this work

A catalogue record for this book
is available from the British Library

ISBN 0 7225 2953 8

Typeset by Harper Phototypesetters Limited
Northampton, England

Printed in Great Britain by
HarperCollinsManufacturing Glasgow

Contents

Note to reader

Before following the self-help advice given in this book, readers are earnestly urged to give careful consideration to the nature of their particular health problem, and to consult a competent physician if in any doubt. This book should not be regarded as a substitute for professional medical treatment, and whilst every care is taken to ensure the accuracy of the content, the author and publishers cannot accept legal responsibility for any problem arising out of the experimentation with the methods described.

PART ONE

Causes

CHAPTER ONE

Why Do Some People Have Bad Breath?

Bad breath is a very widespread problem and one that causes a great deal of embarrassment and personal distress. It impairs relationships, makes working situations difficult and can become a social barrier that leads to isolation and frustration. It can occur at any age, even in young children.

Bad breath is not a disease but may be the result of any of a wide range of underlying health problems, including gum, tooth and mouth cond- itions, sinus and breathing problems, digestive disturbances of many sorts, diabetes and general toxicity. Or its cause may be as simple as a lack of common-sense mouth hygiene – regular cleaning of the teeth or dentures. In some cases it may be the result of something as potentially serious as a liver disease. But more commonly it is caused by health conditions such as a lack of particular digestive enzymes, a chronic sinus, tooth, gum or mouth infection, or a tendency towards constipation.

A series of questionnaires in the next chapter will

help to identify the possible causes in any given case.

One of the problems with halitosis (bad breath's scientific name) is that the person affected may not be aware of the unpleasant odour coming from their mouth every time they breathe out or speak – or if they are, they may not be aware of just how unpleasant it is for those with whom they are in close contact. If they do realise that the condition exists they might well spend a small fortune masking it with mouthwashes, gargles, scented sweets and chewing gums, while not dealing with the underlying causes. As with any health disturbance it is far better to deal with basic causes. This is clearly going to be more effective in the long run than just trying to disguise what is happening.

What's to be done? The good news is that once the causes are identified, remedies to deal with them – and therefore to help eliminate bad breath – are not difficult to discover or to implement. There are some general health tips that can be used by everyone, as well as some specific guidelines that will apply only to some people whose particular requirements they fit.

THE IMPORTANCE OF NUTRITION

Because supplements are going to be recommended later in this book for a number of conditions, we need to address a very vexed question.

Why should some people have different nutritional requirements from others? The recommended daily allowance (RDA) of any particular vitamin or mineral is set by a panel of scientific advisers to governments and is thought by them to meet the essential needs of all 'healthy people'. Are you one of the 'healthy people' whose nutritional needs would be met by taking the RDA suggested by the Department of Health (or the FDA in the USA)?

Even if it is accepted that the RDA is accurate for healthy people (and this is strongly contested by many nutrionists who believe it to be inadequately low in most cases), the list of those who do not fit into the category of essentially healthy people is very long. You might well be in one or more categories, which means that you require additional nutritional support beyond what you get from your food in order to maintain health. You need nutritional supplements if you:

- have a very large or very small body size
- live in a hot climate or work in a hot environment
- are under stress at work
- have wounds, burns, or other injuries
- are taking prescribed medication
- have digestive problems
- are pregnant or a nursing mother
- have an unusual or unique metabolism
- have a chronic illness
- are involved in regular heavy exercise (training, aerobics, etc.)

- regularly consume alcohol or smoke
- regularly consume coffee
- are involved in regular dieting or slimming
- are past retirement age
- are going through puberty
- use oral contraceptives
- have infections
- have too little or no exercise
- are exposed to radiation (even sun-bathing)
- consume polluted water i.e. most tap-water
- are exposed to polluted air or pesticides
- are under emotional stress

And if you do not fit into one of these categories there is another unhappy fact to absorb – that detailed surveys of almost all population groups (young children, school children, teenagers, young adults, the middle-aged and the elderly) in all socio-economic groups regularly show that between 80 per cent and 90 per cent *fail to receive in their daily diet all the RDA of essential nutrients.*

And all of this comes on top of the established fact that before we even start to consider the individual circumstances listed above we *all* begin with different nutritional requirements because of genetic programming. This is known medically as 'biochemical individuality' and it means that in the case of each of the nearly 50 different nutrients (vitamins, minerals, etc.) that we need in order to survive in good health, there will be variations in need from person to person by as much as 700 per cent. Nutritionists and naturopaths find that in most cases of ill health some dietary adjustment, and often supplementation, is needed to help recovery. So when we consider bad breath, which can have a number of underlying health disturbances at its base, nutrition takes a prominent position.

There may also be specific local hygiene strategies that will help, and in all cases attention to common-sense health guidelines will boost overall well-being as well as helping get rid of this unpleasant condition.

Our first task is to look at the possible causes so that you can identify the background to halitosis if it affects you or someone you wish to help.

A word of caution is needed: don't expect results to be immediate if the problem has been around for months or years. In most cases improvement should become apparent within weeks if the causes are identified and appropriate action is started, whether this involves hygienic practices, nutritional changes or more specific health-enhancing strategies. Where causes are not serious or too chronic, complete elimination of halitosis is usually possible within a matter of months. If the cause lies in more chronic imbalances or if there are serious health problems such as liver disease or diabetes, there are likely to be improvements, although they may be slow in coming and perhaps not total.

CHAPTER TWO

Some Causes of Bad Breath

There are some obvious breath odours that result from eating foods such as garlic and which are quite acceptable to some people and absolutely unacceptable to others. This is partly a cultural matter – certain smells are appreciated and not disliked (or are even liked) in one society while being absolutely hated in another. Whatever we eat and drink influences what is carried on the breath, not always from the stomach but often because the lungs are used as a means of elimination of waste products. Particularly strong odours such as onion and garlic will find their way into the stale air we breathe out, some hours after digestion when the food has been broken down and absorbed into the bloodstream. This sort of breath odour is not halitosis, it is simply the end result of what you have eaten or drunk, or of course what you have smoked.

There are many other possible causes to consider when looking for the reasons for real halitosis, which is a distinctly unpleasant odour coming from the mouth.

Be suspicious of having bad breath. Ask people directly whether it is the case, especially if you notice that people avoid getting too close when you are speaking to them, or that they seem to pull away or keep their distance in a social or work situation where others stay close to each other. Ask someone you trust – they may have wanted to tell you for ages but were afraid to do so in case they hurt your feelings.

Once you have identified that the problem exists you have taken a first step towards putting it right. The next stage is to pin-point the cause(s) of the bad breath.

INADEQUATE MOUTH HYGIENE

Of all the likely origins of this socially unpleasant problem there is one that is the simplest to remedy and also the likeliest candidate for the 'main cause' – inadequate brushing and general hygiene of the mouth and teeth. If halitosis is coming from the mouth itself, and if there is no disease of the gums and teeth, then the introduction of regular brushing, flossing and tongue cleansing – after every meal if possible – as well as scrupulous hygiene regarding toothbrushes can often dramatically improve matters.

Bacterial activity, especially when particular

foods such as sugar are eaten, can rapidly reduce the alkalinity of the mouth, encouraging yet more bacterial growth. This can be helped by brushing and flossing and/or the use of medicated toothpicks, which massage the gum between the teeth. Which methods are best is discussed and advice as to the best ways of cleaning teeth and gums is given in chapter 4.

If dentures or orthodontic or prosthetic appliances (braces to correct and straighten teeth in children, for example) are worn then these, along with toothbrushes, need regular cleansing to avoid the build-up of bacterial and fungal activity that can encourage both mouth odour and gum or mouth infection.

Questionnaire

1 Do you clean your teeth at least twice a day (after every meal is best) using an appropriate brush and paste or powder?
2 Every time (or almost every time) you clean your teeth do you spend not less than three minutes doing so?
3 When you clean your teeth do you do so methodically, making sure that both sides of, and the spaces alongside, each tooth are accessed, and that the brushing is both up and down and circular?
4 Do you use a cleansing mouthwash as well as cleaning your teeth?

5 Do you floss daily?

6 Do you regularly (after each meal is best) use medicated wooden toothpicks to cleanse between the teeth and massage the gums?

7 If you have dentures, or wear a removable orthodontic brace, do you ensure that this is cleaned after each meal and thoroughly disinfected daily?

NOTE

In an ideal world all the answers should be 'YES'. Wherever there is a 'NO' answer you are urged to seriously consider changing your habits.

PERIODONTAL (GUM) INFECTIONS AND DISEASE

When the term 'periodontal disease' is used it means that the tissues around the teeth – the gums – are in some way affected. This is a common cause of bad breath.

When the gums themselves are inflamed or infected the condition is called gingivitis, and this commonly results from the accumulation of deposits of a mixture of food particles, bacteria and mucus known as plaque. As plaque develops it causes the gums to swell and bleed, and areas for more plaque deposits form.

Dietary habits that include too much 'soft' food and not enough crisp and gently abrasive food (apples and raw carrots, for example) are one contributory factor, although there can be others, including poor brushing methods as well as the presence of fillings that aggravate the surrounding gum tissue.

Nutritional imbalances and deficiencies are also often involved in this sort of problem, with deficiency of vitamin C, vitamin A, calcium, zinc, folic acid and vitamin B3, as well as low levels of digestive acids, all being possible causes.

Once gingivitis becomes chronic and infected gum disease is established, it is called pyorrhoea. Halitosis is one of its major symptoms. Pyorrhoea can be a by-product of all or any of the following: poor dental hygiene (brushing, flossing, etc.), unbalanced nutrition (a high-sugar diet that is poor in nutrients such as those listed above), chronic ill health such as diabetes, excessive alcohol consumption and smoking. Natural treatment methods for gingivitis and pyorrhoea will be found in chapter 5.

Questionnaire

1 Do your gums usually bleed when you clean your teeth?
2 Are your gums spongy, swollen, sensitive and/or receding?

3 Have you recently (in the last year or two) had gum infections that needed treatment by a dentist or doctor?

NOTE

If you answer 'YES' to any of these you may already have periodontal disease and should see a dentist and/or a dental hygienist as soon as possible, as well as following the guidelines given in chapters 4 and 5 relating to dental health.

MOUTH AND THROAT INFECTION OR INFLAMMATION

Allergies and deficiencies, mechanical injuries caused by biting the cheek, jagged teeth, poorly fitting dentures or orthodontic braces, mouth breathing and alteration in the normal acid/alkaline balance of the mouth because of dietary habits or other illnesses (diabetes, for example) can all lead to the mouth becoming infected by bacteria, viruses, spirochetes or fungi. Such irritations and infections lead almost certainly to mouth odour and natural treatment methods for this are outlined in Chapter 6.

In some cases mouth infections result from the taking of particular medications. They can also result from an interaction between the mercury in fillings of teeth and the mouth tissues in some people.

When the mouth is affected the condition is known as stomatitis, and when the tongue is the problem it is called glossitis. If the tonsils are infected there is usually a degree of bad breath accompanying the condition, and an outline of a safe treatment plan is given in chapter 6.

Questionnaire

1 Do you have mouth ulcers or white thrush patches on the inner cheeks or tongue?
2 Do you have a habit of 'chewing' the inside of your cheeks?
3 Does your tongue have sore, ulcerated or painful patches or spots?
4 Is your mouth (or tongue) very sensitive to temperature variations in food?
5 Do you have teeth, dentures, a bridge or a brace that irritate any part of the soft tissues of the mouth?
6 Is there any recent history of tonsillitis?

NOTE

If any of these questions is answered by 'YES' then consider carefully the advice given in chapter 6 for improving the health of your mouth. Advice from a qualified health-care provider such as a naturopath or homoeopath as well as a visit to your regular medical adviser would also be a good idea.

SINUS INFECTION

Infection or inflammation of the nasal sinuses can be caused by bacteria, fungal and viral organisms. When chronic infection and congestion of the sinuses exists there is frequently a degree of post-nasal drip in which material passes down the back of the throat. An offensive odour can be a feature of such a condition.

Other causes of chronic congestion of this area include the growth of polyps (wart-like structures) or an injury that deforms the nasal cavities and bones. Smoking and chemical substances, as well as allergic conditions, which constantly irritate the delicate mucous membrane of the region, are other possible causes.

When the sinuses are the source of bad breath this can usually be detected by smelling the difference between the breath leaving the mouth and that leaving the nose when you exhale through one or the other.

Other symptoms are usually present when chronic sinusitis exists and the questions in this section will help to identify whether or not this is a feature of someone's halitosis. Natural methods of treatment are given in chapter 7. They involve a range of possible tactics including nutritional changes, the use of herbs and local hydrotherapy (water therapy).

Questionnaire

1 Sinusitis symptoms include headaches, earache, facial pain, reduced sense of smell, and extreme tenderness on the cheekbones, alongside the nose and on the lower forehead around the eyebrows. Do any of these symptoms apply to you regularly?

2 Have you been treated by your doctor for sinus infection?

3 Do you regularly suffer from post-nasal drip, causing you to have to clear your throat or lightly cough frequently?

4 Does your speaking voice have a nasal sound, as though you have a cold or blocked nose?

5 Are your cheekbone areas or the areas below your eyes 'puffy' most of the time?

6 If you regularly produce mucus from the nose or throat is it dark in colour – yellow, brown or green?

7 If you have mucus is it usually clear and watery?

8 Do you have dark circles below the eyes?

9 Do you have a history of injury to the face or nose?

NOTE

'YES' answer to questions 1, 2, 3, 4 or 5 indicate a possible link between bad breath and sinus problems. A 'YES' to question 3 indicates either allergy or infection resulting in excess mucus production. A 'YES' answer to questions 7 or 8 suggests allergy as a possible feature of the condition, while a 'YES' to question 6 indicates infection as the cause of the post-nasal drip. If question 9 is answered positively there could be a mechanical reason for a nasal/sinus obstruction.

MOUTH BREATHING

Most of us wake in the morning with bad breath if we sleep with our mouths open – a common habit, particularly among people who snore and when the nasal passages are blocked for one reason or another, as in sinus infection or allergy problems. When mouth breathing is habitual during the day as well, bad breath is far more pronounced. If the causes of mouth breathing can be corrected the habit can be broken.

Questionnaire

1 Are you a mouth breather?
2 Do you snore?

NOTE

There are many possible causes of mouth breathing and the advice in chapter 8 should help to correct many of these and therefore the bad breath that results. Improved general health reduces snoring habits.

LIVER DISEASE

Liver disease resulting from alcohol and/or drug abuse, chemical exposure, malnutrition or infection will usually have bad breath as a symptom. The liver is the main detoxification organ of your body and careful dietary and general health care can help a sick liver to recover. *However, if there is a liver problem expert advice is essential*. Advice is given in chapter 9 for detoxification as well as general support for the liver using diet and herbs.

What we eat and drink, as well as the chemicals to which we are exposed (including medication), along with our inherited genetic weaknesses and strengths decide how well we, and our liver, can cope. Chiropractor and naturopath Boris Chaitow has encapsulated in one paragraph all that is wrong with modern diet, in *My Health Secrets* (C. W. Daniel & Co., 1982).

Humans evolved in distant history on a diet of fruits, nuts, whole cereals, plants, herbs and possibly small animals – all nutritionally whole and all rich in the essential nutrients the body requires for high efficiency, energy and freedom from disease – especially the amino acids, mineral salts, trace elements, vitamin and enzymes. Today's human is the only creature on the planet which has deliberately corrupted its source of nourishment. If you think this an exaggeration consider the modern diet – excessively rich in animal proteins, cooked rich and fatty – high levels of starches derived in the main from refined ingredients including white bread, buns, cakes, cookies, puddings, pies as well as white sugar, sweets, chocolates, preserves and jellies, cooked refined and processed cereals, polished rice and ice-cream along with fluids from tea, coffee, cocoa, alcohol and synthetic and artificially sweetened soft drinks – fried, pickled, preserved, cured, smoked, salted and tinned meats and fish – dairy products which are pasteurized and distorted by over-concentrated extractions – with food doctored by colouring, flavouring, preserving, sweetening, salting, chemicalising and overcooking to create foodless materials which contribute to the noxious encumbrances and deficiencies largely responsible for today's tragic state of ill-health. In laboratory experiments such 'foods' cause rats to lose their hair and teeth, to abort their young, to become irritable, pugnacious and cannabalistic – and in ludicrous seriousness causes humans to become pouchy, grouchy, with falling hair, rotting teeth, poached-egg eyes, toxic bowels, pickled livers, bleeding piles and with no idea of what eating or health is all about. And bad breath!

Questionnaire

1 Have you ever been treated for liver disease?
2 Have you in the past consumed, or do you currently consume, excessive levels of alcohol (more than is commonly thought of as safe)?
3 Have you been regularly or heavily exposed to toxic chemicals such as carbon tetrachloride of chloroform?
4 Do you have difficulty in digesting fatty foods or carbohydrates?

NOTE

Liver disease is serious and requires expert medical care. If you have a past history of such problems there may be a lot you can do to help this vital organ to function more efficiently. If you are still abusing your liver through alcohol or chemical exposure this should be stopped as soon as possible. Safe methods to help the liver when it is under stress from such irritants will be found in chapter 9. If you have difficulty in digesting certain food (question 4) there may be factors other than the liver responsible, and the attention to diet and appropriate supplementation of enzymes should help (see chapter 10).

The chances of liver disease being responsible for bad breath are not as great as the likelihood that it derives from poor mouth hygiene or periodontal disease; but if you have a history that suggests liver involvement this could be the cause of unpleasant mouth tastes and odours. This should be addressed by a suitably qualified adviser.

DIGESTIVE PROBLEMS

If lifestyle and diet are unbalanced a range of digestive problems can result. Bad breath may be a symptom of this due to inadequate breakdown of the food eaten.

Once food is consumed it should rapidly (within a matter of a few hours) pass from the stomach into the intestines for further processing. If this movement is sluggish, or the breakdown of the food is poor, putrefaction occurs and the gas from this has to pass either up or down the digestive tract. If the gas is eliminated by belching the breath will of course be tainted.

Attention to what is eaten and how it is eaten (adequate chewing, for example), along with the best combinations of different foods, can all help such problems. Food sensitivity or allergy, digestive acid and/or digestive enzyme deficiencies (or more rarely, excessive levels of acid), lack of adequate fibre and even inadequate exercise can all play a part in producing poor digestion.

Guidelines are given in chapter 10 for digestive problems that are identified as part of the background to bad breath.

Questionnaire

1 Do you chew your food thoroughly until it becomes paste-like?
2 Do you avoid drinking liquids with your meals?
3 Do you eat fresh fruit, vegetables and/or salad most days?
4 Do you regularly (each day) eat fried food, fatty foods, white sugar or red meat products?
5 Do you suffer from indigestion, acidity, bloating or heartburn more than once a week?

NOTE

The answers to questions 1, 2 and 3 should of course be 'YES' and if they are not it is up to you to change your habits to make the most of the chance for better digestion.

The answers to questions 4 and 5 should hopefully be 'NO', but if they were both 'YES', you can modify habits to change 4, and this (along with attention to questions 1, 2 and 3) might well be enough to help you change the answer to question 5 to a 'NO'. If this is not sufficient to improve digestion look at chapter 10 for further advice.

CONSTIPATION

If bowel movements are sluggish the chances of putrefaction increase, as does the likelihood of absorption into the bloodstream of toxic breakdown products, which can then find their way onto the breath via the lungs. Bad breath is a common feature of constipation, although medically it is not generally accepted as a cause. Nevertheless, experience seems to prove that once constipation is relieved, breath sweetness often returns . A combination of dietary reform, exercise and use of appropriate herbs can usually improve this situation. Strategies are outlined in chapter 11.

Questionnaire

1 Do you have a bowel movement at least once daily?

2 Is the bowel movement achieved without strain?

NOTE

Unless both these questions are answered with 'YES' you need to pay attention to your bowel function. Advice that will help in this direction will be found in chapter 11.

BAD BREATH AS A SYMPTOM OF SPECIFIC DISEASE

Just as alcohol on the breath is easy to smell when someone has consumed sufficient to become intoxicated, so there can appear other odours relating to a wide range of health problems. The breath of people with diabetes mellitus, for example, often has a sweet, fruity smell resulting from acetone in the breath. When this is severe it is often possible to recognise it as soon as the person enters a room. The same acetone breath is also present in other conditions, for example in young children who because they are ill have not eaten for a day or so. Similar breath odours are common when people fast for religious or health reasons as the body begins to burn fats for energy.

In advanced kidney disease, when there is urine in the blood (uraemia), a strong ammonia smell is often noticed on the breath. Some forms of liver disease (parenchymal disease) produce an amine smell that is 'musty' and is often used as a diagnostic sign by doctors.

As mentioned above there is also a characteristic disagreeable smell resulting from infection in the mouth, whether this is in the gums or teeth or in the form of sores (ulcers) in the mouth. One of the most unpleasant odours on the breath results from gangrene in the lung, smelling as it does of decaying vegetable matter – the result of the activity of particular bacteria. Finally, some drugs such as those containing iodine, bismuth, turpentine, paraldehyde or creosote, give a characteristic odour to the breath.

If you suspect that you have diabetes or other serious health condition you should see a doctor as soon as possible. If you are already receiving attention for such a condition and have bad breath consult your medical adviser before adopting any of the advice given in this book. If you suspect your bad breath results from periodic fasting or from a mouth condition you should follow the advice in this book as well as considering taking other expert advice.

NO SPECIFIC ADVICE IS GIVEN IN THIS BOOK RELATING TO THE SORT OF BAD BREATH ASSOCIATED WITH KIDNEY DISEASE OR DIABETES, AS THESE CONDITIONS REQUIRE EXPERT MEDICAL

ADVICE RATHER THAN SELF-TREATMENT. AGAIN, DO NOT ADOPT ANY OF THE ADVICE GIVEN IN THIS BOOK WITHOUT CONSULTING YOUR MEDICAL ADVISER IF YOU HAVE SUCH A CONDITION.

COMBINATIONS OF CAUSES

In many cases of halitosis there is a combination of causes, and all need to be dealt with for a happy solution to this anti-social problem. Inadequate diet, poor digestion, poor dental or gum hygiene and health, constipation, catarrh and sinus congestion and/or infection, and possible food allergies or sensitivities, often accompanied by mouth breathing, may all be present and in need of attention. Fortunately none of these are 'serious' and all can usually be helped, mainly by attention to basic nutrition and lifestyle habits.

CHAPTER THREE

First Aid for Bad Breath

Having seen the many possible causes of bad breath it must be clear that in some cases it is going to take a good deal of effort and dedication in order to normalise the health problems that may lie behind the bad breath. In many cases the solution is reasonably easy, a simple matter of applying common-sense mouth-hygiene. In other cases, however, there may be long-standing mouth, throat, sinus or digestive problems resulting from allergy, deficiency, toxicity or infection, which need to be sorted out before the breath is going to be as sweet as it can and should be.

While such efforts are being undertaken there is obviously room for first aid to help improve the situation, and there is an abundance of commercial products that can be sprayed, swallowed, chewed or in some other way used to mask bad breath. Most are reasonably harmless, if somewhat chemical, in their actions. The advice given below for first aid suggests a number of more natural products and methods, many of which also have positive, health-enhancing benefits to offer. This is seldom the case with commercial mouth-freshening products.

The danger always exists that if symptoms are masked, disguised or hidden, the cause might be neglected. This can prove to be a costly mistake, largely because like any other symptom bad breath is a sign that all is not well somewhere and if this sign is neglected the problem can become worse. If the causes of bad breath are not dealt with the end result could be as serious as the loss of teeth as the gum condition deteriorates. So when applying first aid measures for bad breath, make sure that you also take up the challenge that the condition poses and sort out the background causes as well.

FIRST AID OPTIONS

- From a health store obtain a source of chlorophyll in the form of alfalfa, barley or wheatgrass juice and drink a tablespoon of this two or three times a day.
- Add a teaspoon of such a juice to a half a tumbler of water and use this as a mouthwash several times daily – on waking and on going to bed at the very least.
- Obtain essential oil of cloves (any pharmacy or health store) and add two drops to a tumbler of water and use as a mouthwash as often as you wish through the day.
- Obtain French fine green (or white superfine) clay and stir a teaspoonful into a tumbler of pure (not tap)

water and drink this between meals twice daily. Clay has profound detoxification effects as the clay passes through you taking toxins with it.

- Use a clay solution (two teaspoonsful in a tumbler of water) as a mouthwash. Try to retain the water in your mouth as long as possible for local detoxification effects.
- From a herbal supplier, oriental food store or health store obtain fennel seeds, cardamom and/or anise seeds and chew these after meals and throughout the day whenever you become aware of your mouth not having a sweet taste.
- Place a clove in your mouth and gently suck or chew it as a breath freshener.
- Chew parsley leaves (fresh or dried) for mouth freshness as often as you feel the need – and especially after a garlic-rich meal!
- Instead of regular tea, drink chamomile or peppermint tea, especially if indigestion is a feature.
- If you have a juice extractor, once or twice daily drink a mixture of carrot and celery juice (include parsley and alfalfa if you can).
- Eat fresh fruit whenever you are peckish – an apple several times daily is good for the teeth, gums and digestion.
- Clean your teeth with clay toothpaste and chew clay gum (from specialist health stores – see Resources section) for additional detoxification of the mouth.
- Homoeopathic remedies can be used safely to deal with bad breath relating to the following situations (the author wishes to thank Weleda for their help in compiling this list):

If the breath is sour due to indigestion and acidity use the homoeopathic remedy Nux vomica 6C, two or three times a day for up to a week. Note: these dosages and frequencies are the same for all the remedies listed below. This remedy is most appropriate if the problem is worse after meals, if there is also slight nausea, if it is worse in the morning or after drinking alcohol.

If the breath is strongly offensive, and there is a lot of saliva, a degree of dental decay and the tongue is yellow and furred, use Merc. sol. 6C.

If the breath is foul after eating fatty food and the mouth is dry without a feeling of thirst, use Pulsatilla 6C.

If the breath is putrid or bitter in a young person around the age of puberty, use Aurum met. 6C.

If the breath smells of garlic or onions, use Petroleum 6C or Asafoetida 6C or Sinapsis nigra 6C.

If there has been an injury and bleeding in the mouth and the bad breath relates to this, use Arnica 6C.

If after sleep the mouth is coated with mucus and a bad breath accompanies this, use Rheum 6C.

For bad breath that accompanies constipation, use Acidum carbolicum 6C.

For bad breath accompanied by palpitations, use Spigelia 6C.

If the breath smells like rotten cheese, use Mazereum 6C.

If the breath smells like urine, use Graphites 6C.

These homoeopathic remedies are available from good health stores, many pharmacies and direct from specialist suppliers – see Resources section.

PART TWO

Treatment

CHAPTER FOUR

Essential Oral Hygiene

Plaque is a material that is made in the mouth, mainly out of food particles and bacteria. It is the main cause of dental and gum disease, which is itself one of the main reasons for bad breath. The bacteria that help manufacture plaque – it takes between 12 and 24 hours to form – love sugars of all sorts, and when they use this for food they produce acids as a by-product. It is the acids that cause the damage to the teeth and gums.

One of the first and most important tasks in preventing or eliminating bad breath is dealing with plaque. There are some simple rules that can help to improve dental, gum and mouth health and also reduce the chances of infection of the gums and mouth.

BRUSHING

Brush your teeth after every meal and on rising and

at bedtime. If this is not always possible brush them at least twice a day and also use some other method to clean the spaces between the teeth after meals.

When brushing try to use strokes that are mainly downwards when cleaning the upper teeth and upwards when cleaning the lower teeth, so that your brush moves from gum to tooth. To clean under the gums, where plaque forms, angle the brush so that the bristles are facing upwards and back for the upper front gums and downwards and back for the lower front gums. They should face upwards and forwards and downwards and forwards for the upper and lower inside gums. Holding the brush in this way use *very short* strokes (and a very soft brush) to massage and cleanse all the gum edges. When cleaning the back teeth use circular motions on their flat surfaces.

The problem with the toothbrush is its limitation in getting into all the spaces between the teeth, where gum problems usually start. For this task you need to floss or use a suitable toothpick.

FLOSSING

Flossing the teeth to remove particles between the teeth or between the teeth and gums should be performed immediately before or after brushing for best effects.

There are various forms of floss – some are waxed, others are not and some are more like a tape (known as dental tape) than a fine string. Which should you use? The waxed versions leave a film on the teeth which protects them – this is not suitable if there is regular painting of the teeth with protective substances such as fluoride. If there are a lot of fillings with rough surfaces the tape may be easier to use than the floss.

You may need to get advice from a dental hygienist as to the best ways of flossing; however, there are some general guidelines that can be helpful.

1 Be slow and methodical (don't skip any areas) for the best results.
2 Use about six to nine inches of floss or tape, creating a loop by tying the ends together. Hold the loop in each hand and gently insert the floss or tape between two teeth. Pull it back and forwards between the teeth and also wrap it around a tooth taking it to the place where the tooth meets the gum. Move it up and down and gently around the teeth, using both hands – this will loosen the plaque.
3 Don't be so vigorous as to cause bleeding or discomfort – just allow the tape or floss to press hard enough on the gum for you to be aware of it.

TOOTHPICKS

Similar results to flossing can be achieved by using medicated wooden toothpicks, available from pharmacists. These are used to massage the gums lightly and clean away food debris and plaque. Gently apply the tip of the pick to the groove where the gum and tooth meet and clean the surface of the tooth. This is most useful in the area of the inner aspects of the lower teeth and the outer (cheek-side) aspects of the upper back teeth.

MOUTHWASH

A mouthwash that promotes oral hygiene, eliminating undesirable micro-organisms and soothing tender gums and mucous membrane should be used every day.

TONGUE CLEANSING

Daily tongue cleansing is a great help in promoting mouth health. Gently scrape the surface debris off the tongue using a spoon or wooden spatula and then rinse thoroughly with a safe mouthwash. Gentle brushing of the tongue with a soft tooth-brush can also be effective before rinsing.

THE TOOTHBRUSH

Use only soft toothbrushes for your teeth, gums and tongue, and change the brush every month to six weeks.

Make sure the brush is thoroughly disinfected everyday as the bristles and brush-head can become colonised by bacteria or fungi. There are special sanitising machines to help kill these organisms, or you can leave the brush to soak in a mild disinfectant, washing it well before and after each use.

TOOTHPASTES

Many toothpastes contain undesirable substances that can irritate the gums, such as the detergent lauryl sulphate, bleaching agents, and artificial colouring and flavouring. Many of these can trigger sensitivity or allergic responses in the mouth. Alternative substances for use in brushing and mouth washing include:

- bicarbonate of soda and sea salt, which some manufacturers have combined in a paste, or which you can mix yourself
- products that include herbal extracts, clay and various bark extracts, which have traditional use as dental aids.

There is a wide variety of natural products used in toothpastes, mouthwashes, chewing gums and mouth-freshening sprays including combinations of herbs (rosemary, echinacea, tea tree, myrrh, sage, fennel, peppermint, cinnamon), French clay (which has powerful detoxification qualities), homoeopathic ingredients, various tree barks and propolis as well as calcium and fluoride. Manufacturers from all over the world are involved in production of this array of dental health products – details of which are to be found in the resources section on page 101.

There are many other excellent dental products free of the chemicals and the excessively abrasive substances used in commercial pastes and powders. These include various Japanese seaweed toothpastes; peelu, a tree-derived substance from the Middle East and Asia; and meswak, another tree extract, which has anti-inflammatory and antibiotic properties.

DENTURES

If you wear dentures, a removable bridge or a brace (orthodontic) then these need to be thoroughly cleaned and disinfected every single day. Studies have shown that when this is not done a reservoir of infectious organisms, including yeasts and bacteria, can develop. This can lead to constant reinfection of the mouth and gums. The dentures or brace should be soaked in a disinfectant solution every night and well brushed to remove all traces of food particles or plaque.

HOME PREPARATIONS

There are a number of do-it-yourself ways of preparing and using herbal and other mouthwashes to enhance dental and oral health.

1 Buy fennel or anise seeds from a health store or herbal supplier and munch these several times daily, especially after meals.

2 Use diluted aloe vera juice (several dessertspoonsful in a tumbler of water) as a mouthwash. Sip a little, rinsing the mouth and spitting out, and then drink the remainder, allowing the liquid good contact with all aspects of your mouth before swallowing. Aloe vera is antibiotic, antifungal and soothing.

3 Chew parsley leaves as often as you can during the day for their detoxifying effect on the mouth. This also masks garlic smells.

4 Chew crunchy foods throughout the day – apples, carrots and celery are good as these remove plaque and cleanse the teeth naturally. Avoid sugary foods such as cakes, biscuits and, especially, sweets.

SUMMARY

Clean your teeth or dentures daily, after meals and morning and evening, using appropriate materials; use flossing and/or toothpick and mouthwash routines to further cleanse the mouth and tongue, while maintaining hygienic routines regarding the brush you use. Take care over what you eat and drink.

These mouth hygiene tips are vital if you are going to overcome bad breath. Start today to apply those not already part of your routine, and stick to your determination to overcome the problem.

CHAPTER FIVE

Gum Disease

When only the gums are inflamed the condition is known as gingivitis, and this can be an acute or chronic condition. Once it becomes chronic, inflammation of the tissues that support the teeth can also occur and this is called periodontal disease. Bad breath is likely to be present with both gingivitis and periodontal disease.

When there is periodontal disease the gums will be swollen, sensitive and will bleed easily. The gums may also be receding leaving the lower margins of the teeth exposed and sensitive to heat, cold and acids. Periodontal problems are more frequent in puberty and pregnancy, possibly due to hormonal changes, and are commonly associated with allergy, heavy metal (lead, mercury, cadmium, etc.) toxicity as well as with diabetes and nutritional deficiency conditions.

Self-help methods should start with application of the various guidelines and tips suggested in the previous pages relating to mouth hygiene and the removal of plaque and tartar (plaque deposits that have become concreted when mixed with saliva). As well as trying to help the condition yourself such problems should also be under the supervision of a dentist and hygienist for best results, and a twice yearly (at least) visit to such a health professional is suggested.

Much of the advice in this section regarding nutrition is based on verifiable medical studies, as outlined in Professor Melvyn Werbach's book *Nutritional Influences on Illness* (Third Line Press, 1992). There are books that recommend far higher doses of the nutrients listed below, and such levels may well be appropriate in some cases of periodontal and other diseases. However, I believe that such levels of supplementation should be used only under professional guidance. The doses recommended below are safe for self-use and should prove helpful in most cases.

EATING HABITS

Your diet should include as much in the way of *whole foods* as possible (whole grains, brown rice, unrefined foods) and it is best to avoid sugary foods such as cakes, biscuits and sweets.

Food should be as 'chewy' as possible since soft mushy foods do not encourage chewing, with the result that gums do not get the stimulation, exercise and 'massage' that helps to reduce the swelling and irritation present in periodontal disease. For this reason as many servings daily as possible of fresh fruit – particularly the berries and grapes for their vitamin, enzyme and mineral content, as well as crisp, crunchy fruits such as apples, for their direct cleansing and gum-stimulating influence – should be included in the diet, along with salads and raw or lightly cooked vegetables. Above all, recommendation number one is avoid sugar.

Supplementation

A number of nutrients are commonly deficient in people with gum and periodontal disease and these can be usefully supplemented to help the condition (and so help reduce bad breath), while some such as folic acid, zinc and vitamin E can also be applied to the irritated tissues directly or used in a mouthwash.

FOLIC ACID

This B vitamin is commonly lacking in modern diets and anyone using contraceptive medication (the Pill) is likely to be deficient in it. Taking 1 milligram daily of folic acid, or using a mouthwash solution containing 0.1 per cent folic acid, has been shown to help the health of inflamed gums significantly. In one study when the solution was used, the mouth was rinsed for a minute twice daily and improvement was seen within two weeks.

VITAMIN A

Deficiency of vitamin A is known to predispose towards periodontal disease and a supplement that includes it would be helpful, as would inclusion in the diet of foods rich in vitamin A or beta carotene (which becomes vitamin A in the body), such as green, yellow and orange vegetables and fruits.

This vitamin is especially needed during times of actual gum infection, at which time high doses (up to 25,000IU daily) should be taken for three or four days followed by a maintenance dosage of around 10,000IU daily. Also drink carrot juice or eat melons regularly for their beta carotene.

VITAMIN C

A standard question to discover possible vitamin C deficiency is 'Do your gums bleed when you clean your teeth?' Bacterial toxins are prevented from infiltrating the mucous membrane of the mouth when vitamin C is in plentiful supply, and so fresh fruits and vegetables, rich in C, as well as supplementation of the vitamin is a good idea when there is active periodontal disease. A supplemental dose of 500 to 1000 milligrams daily of vitamin C (ideally in a form that contains bioflavonoids) is suggested.

Many people take higher levels of vitamin C and it is quite safe to do so. There are *no* toxic side-effects from vitamin C supplementation. The only slightly negative thing that might happen when extremely high levels are consumed is mild, harmless diarrhoea. The levels suggested above are probably enough to help normalise deficiency levels in most people with gum problems and will not cause diarrhoea.

VITAMIN E

Studies show that when the gums are inflamed it is helpful once a day to break an 800 mg vitamin E capsule, and to swish the oil around the mouth, rubbing it gently into the gums, before swallowing. One medical study showed that after three weeks of doing this there was a distinct improvement in inflamed tissues compared with results in a group of people who did the same thing with dummy capsules.

COMBINATION

A combination of vitamins A, E and K, taken supplementally and applied locally to inflamed tissues, has been shown to improve the health of periodontal tissues.

CALCIUM

People with periodontal disease (as well as denture wearers) commonly have low calcium intakes.

Supplementing with between a gram and a gram and a half (1000 to 1500 mg) of calcium daily has been shown to reduce the damage that the disease can cause to the bone surrounding the teeth.

MAGNESIUM

This mineral helps the body to use calcium for rebuilding damaged tissues. Tests show that its supplementation can make a huge difference to the restoration of bone loss around teeth in periodontal disease. 500 mg daily is suggested when calcium is being supplemented at 1000 mg daily.

ZINC

Zinc is one of the commonest deficiencies in the industrialised world and lack of it leads to increased damage to gingival (gum) tissues. A combination of supplementation (20 to 30 mg daily) and use of a zinc mouthwash (containing around 25 mM soluble zinc) can help to reduce plaque formation and tissue damage.

COENZYME Q10

Japanese studies show that supplementation of this nutrient (50 mg daily in divided doses) improves the health of inflamed gingival tissues in most people taking it.

Summary of Nutritional Advice

Eat whole food and avoid sugary foods.

Supplement with

- 1 mg daily folic acid
- 10,000IU daily vitamin A
- 500 to 1,000 mg daily vitamin C
- 1 gram daily of calcium
- 500 mg daily of magnesium
- 20 mg daily of zinc
- 50 mg daily of coenzyme Q

Apply topically to the gums all or any of the following

- folic acid mouthwash solution (0.1%)
- vitamin E (break an 800 mg capsule and massage gums with oil)
- zinc mouthwash solution (25 mM soluble zinc)

Herbal and Other Methods

Choose one of the following at a time to combine with the nutritional methods suggested above:

- Paint the gums up to three times daily using a soft paintbrush with a small amount of a mixture of equal parts of tinctures of myrrh and echinacea (from a health store or herbal supplier).
- Use goldenseal herb powder as a tooth powder (i.e. brush with it) for a month to assess its benefits in reducing bleeding gums and inflammation.

- Each morning and every evening mix a tablespoon of apple cider vinegar in a cup of water and use half of it as a mouthwash, and after spitting this out drink the rest.
- Place a little oak bark power (from a herbal supplier) between the gums and the cheeks at night before sleep.
- Homoeopathic assistance for gum inflammation is often gained by taking Kreosotum 6X, available from homoeopathic pharmacies and some health stores.

DIGESTIVE ACID

There is commonly a deficiency of hydrochloric acid production in the stomach when periodontal disease is present, and this should be checked out. See chapter 10 for further information. It is probably the reduction in calcium absorption resulting from poor digestion that influences periodontal problems when hydrochloric acid deficiency exists. The same sort of acid deficiency is common when allergies exist and this may also be a factor with problems in the mouth.

MERCURY TOXICITY

Mercury from the amalgams in filled teeth leaches slowly into the mouth and body and has been shown to be a major factor in some cases of gum disease. Suggestions as to possible strategies to apply to this problem will be found in chapter 6.

CHAPTER SIX

Mouth and Throat Problems

Inflammation of the tissues of the mouth (other than the gums and teeth) can be a cause of bad breath. The possible causes of mouth irritation and inflammation were outlined in chapter 2 on page 13 and these causes need to be identified before specific appropriate self-help measures can be introduced. The causes usually fall into one of four groups: allergy, deficiency, irritation or infection.

ALLERGY

Ulcers in the mouth (aphthous ulcers) and many painful inflammations of the tongue and throat which can lead to bad breath are commonly caused by food allergy, in which case there may well be other symptoms such as fatigue, palpitations, mood swings, muscle aching, indigestion and skin problems. In one study it was found that a quarter of all people with mouth ulcers were wheat sensitive, while in another almost half the people evaluated had sensitivities to either milk, cheese, wheat, tomato, vinegar, lemon, pineapple or mustard.

Identifying Allergies

The allergy may need to be identified by an expert such as a clinical ecologist or a naturopath. There are also ways of doing this yourself by temporary exclusion of particular foods (bread, milk, etc.) or food families (all grains or all dairy products, for example). This is a bit hit-or-miss but can sometimes be effective. One of the strongest clues as to which foods to exclude can be learned by looking at what foods you eat almost every day – and which ones you can't imagine being without. Target such foods for five day eliminations to see what happens to the symptoms of mouth (or other) inflammation or irritation.

Other strategies that can help identify the causes in cases of food allergy are outlined in *Nutritional Medicine* by Drs Alan Stewart and Stephen Davies. One of their suggestions is for a 'pears and lamb diet' in which for five days only pears and lamb (or turkey) are eaten. These two foods are seldom involved in allergy and the five-day period allows the body to clear itself of all previously consumed allergens. If the condition of mouth ulcers (or any other allergy) improves dramatically on this regime it is possible to then begin the slow process of identifying the culprit foods.

No one should stay on a limited pear and lamb diet for more than a week without being under expert supervision.

Another alternative, which allows for more variety, is the so-called 'oligoantigenic diet', which has been widely used to flush out allergens at many medical centres including Great Ormond Street Hospital for Sick Children. On this diet ONLY the following foods can be eaten – again for a short period but this time three weeks is suggested as the safe limit for self-assessment using this less restrictive diet.

The oligoantigenic diet *suggests* that you eat:

- Lamb, turkey, rabbit, lean game
- White fish (not if you have eczema)
- Any vegetables but not potatoes, onions, sweet corn or soya
- Only the following fruits – bananas, mangoes, paw paw, peeled pears, pomegranates
- All cereals but not wheat, oats, barley, rye and corn
- Sunflower oil, safflower oil, olive oil, linseed oil (all others should be avoided)
- Tomor or Vitasieg margarine (avoid all other dairy produce)
- Herbal teas such as camomile – avoid coffee (even decaffeinated) and regular tea
- Distilled or deionised water – avoid all fruit juices, tap-water, alcohol
- Use only sea salt as a condiment – avoid all other spices and salts

- Avoid honey and sugar of all sorts

Whichever method is used, when you have proof that a food or food family is guilty of provoking allergies it should be left out of the diet for some months before an attempt is made to reintroduce it. If it again provokes a reaction then it should be eliminated for at least six moths.

Once culprit foods are identified a system known as the 'rotation diet', in which foods from particular 'families' of foods (dairy or grains for example) are eaten at most once in four days is used by many experts to help prevent constant provocation by allergens in the diet. The details of this excellent approach needs to be carefully explained by a health professional such as a properly qualified health counsellor or a naturopath or a doctor using these methods (usually a clinical ecologist).

DEFICIENCY

When the normal bacterial flora of the mouth are deficient or the acid/alkaline level of the mouth alters for any reason (allergy, deficiency, etc.) this encourages undesirable bacteria to breed and mouth ulcers to form. Supplementation with *Lactobacillus acidophilus* can help this, and studies have shown that regular (once or twice daily) rinsing of the mouth with water in which these 'friendly' bacteria have been mixed speeds up the healing. Brands that contain a large number of viable organisms, such as Natren Superdophilus or BioCare's Bioacidophilus, are best.

Deficiencies of iron, vitamin B12, folic acid or vitamin B6 can all cause mouth ulcerations. Research has shown that in one group of over 300 people with mouth ulcers almost 15 per cent had one or more of these deficiencies. Nearly 90 per cent of these improved, many completely, following supplementation.

Vitamin C deficiency often shows up as tiny areas of bleeding under the tongue or enlargement of the veins under the tongue (bruising after slight bumps is also likely to be noticed with C deficiency). When vitamin C is deficient iron absorption from food usually becomes less efficient and can lead to anaemia, which itself often produces a range of mouth symptoms. If iron or B12 are deficient there would probably also be other symptoms. If iron or B12 are deficient there would probably also be other symptoms such as extreme tiredness, loss of appetite, headaches, constipation, loss of concentration and irritability, as well as a pale appearance and a blue tinge to the white of the eyes. In this case, expert advice should be obtained. Other obvious symptoms of deficiency of vitamin B12, iron or folic acid could include a smooth and painful tongue, and vitamin B12 deficiency also results in cracks at the corner of the mouth.

Taking a vitamin C supplement at meal times (500 mg twice daily) and including plenty of fresh fruit and vegetables in the diet will usually take care of iron deficiency.

When vitamin B2 (riboflavin), B3 (niacin) and B6 (pyridoxine) are deficient a variety of tongue and mouth signs become obvious. The tongue will have cracks and fissures when there is a lack of B3 and prominent enlarged taste buds and/or a red, sore tip with B2 and B6 deficiency. A general supplement of vitamin B complex (any health store or pharmacy) taken for a month or so will usually show whether one of the B vitamins is lacking, although there can be reasons why these are not being adequately absorbed from the diet (such as deficiency of digestive acids and enzymes) which would need expert investigation.

Some cases of mouth ulceration improve when zinc is supplemented although no clear link has been established between deficiency and ulceration.

IRRITATION

Any obvious causes of mouth irritation such as ill-fitting dentures or dental appliances should be dealt with by a dentist.

Only some dentists are currently prepared to investigate and help eliminate the link between excessive mercury fillings and a variety of health problems, including mouth and tongue soreness. Contact the British Dental Society for Clinical

Nutrition (see Resources section) for the name of your nearest such practitioner if you wish to investigate this possibility.

A useful homoeopathic remedy (homoeopathic pharmacy or good health store) for use when the tongue is severely coated in yellow material is Chelidonium 6X. This is taken several times a day away from meals, dissolved in the mouth.

MOUTH INFECTIONS

The commonest mouth infection leading to bad breath involves the yeast *Candida albicans*, and is often called 'thrush'. The symptoms of this are white patches on the inner cheek, gums or tongue, which may be sore. Treating the body as a whole – as opposed to simply treating the local outbreak of infection – will get the best results.

I have a simple but thorough self-help outline for dealing with Candida in my book *Candida Albicans – Could Yeast be Your Problem* (Thorsons, 1991). The following is a basic summary of the best way of starting to get rid of yeast.

Firstly it is necessary to understand that when Candida affects the mouth or throat it is already widely spread in the intestines and possibly the vaginal area. This is why symptoms such as digestive distress (bloating, 'acid' stomach, diarrhoea or constipation) and genito-urinary problems (recurrent cystitis, vaginitis, etc.) are all too common along with mouth and throat infection by yeast. Any local treatment focusing only on the mouth (or vagina) will have limited short term effects, so it is necessary to pay particular attention to the 'reservoir' of yeast that may be flourishing in the bowel.

Everyone has some Candida but it is usually controlled efficiently by the immune system and by huge colonies of friendly bacteria living in our intestinal tracts (including the mouth, which is the start of the intestinal tract) and on our skin. It often gets out of hand, though, when antibiotics and other medication are used too enthusiastically or too often – especially if the diet is unbalanced, with too much sugar and not enough nutrient-rich foods.

An approach that uses a triple attack is usually best in order to avoid a repetitive cycle in which Candida outbreaks occur in the mouth or vagina or elsewhere whenever you are under stress or the immune system is under pressure (with another infection, for example).

This three-pronged approach attempts to kill the yeast by using a variety of herbal products such as garlic, caprylic acid (coconut plant extract), aloe vera juice, Glycyrrhiza (licorice plant), hydrastis and/or echinacea (herbal antibiotics).

At the same time replenishment of bowel flora is started using proven viable colonising strains of Lactobacillus acidophilus (for the mouth, vagina and small intestine) and Bifidobacteria (for the large intestine). These are the normal controlling element for Candida which are usually damaged when antibiotics or steroid drugs (including the Pill) are used medically, allowing the yeast to get out of hand.

In addition a general low sugar/high complex-carbohydrate diet together with cultured (live) dairy products is suggested. Sugar is yeast's favourite food – ask anyone who makes wine or beer – and it makes sense not to feed it while you are trying to kill it with herbs and friendly bacteria.

Such methods are commonly extremely successful but may take six months or more to control the yeast overgrowth completely – although mouth and other local symptoms should show improvement within weeks.

It is all too common for people with Candida to have additional food sensitivities and allergies caused by the activity of the yeast in the intestines – the yeast allows absorption of undesirable substances that trigger the allergy reactions. For this reason extra care over diet is needed, avoiding anything that seems to provoke symptoms, especially if it is itself derived from yeasts or carries moulds on it.

Diet to Candida

Avoid all sugars and for the first few weeks avoid fruit as well. Avoid aged cheeses, dried fruits, any fermented products and any food derived from or containing yeast. Eat at least three ounces daily of fish, poultry or lean meat (free range only as many factory-farmed animals and fish contain antibiotic and steroid residues) unless you are vegetarian, in which case substitute grains and pulses for this. Eat pulses (beans, lentils) and whole grains, especially rice, and abundantly of salad or lightly cooked vegetables. Daily consumption of live cultured milk products (low fat if possible) such as yogurt or kefir is extremely helpful in Candida conditions, but avoid these if you are dairy sensitive. Make sure that such products contain live organisms and no sugar!

Supplements for Controlling Candida

- Caprylic acid (coconut plant extract) capsules – two to four daily with meals.
- Acidophilus and Bifidobacteria (Natren or BioCare brands) – a quarter of a teaspoonful of each (or Biocare capsule) three times daily away from meals.
- Also use acidophilus powder in the mouth each night, directly or dissolved in water.
- Garlic (Kyolic or PureGar brands) – three to six capsules daily.
- Aloe vera juice – one teaspoon in small tumbler of water as a mouthwash and drunk several times a day.
- Echinacea C chewable tablets – several times daily to help control other undesirable mouth and throat organisms.

Additional help from herbs such as licorice or hydrastis requires expert advice.

NOTE

Expect to feel slightly unwell for the first few days of an anti-candida diet as your body has to deal with the dead yeast – you may feel flu-like symptoms or nausea. Be patient and stick to the programme.

If you have any tendency to Candidiasis or other infections in the mouth take extra care over disinfecting toothbrushes and in any case start using a new one at least once a month to prevent reinfection, as brushes are a notorious haven for micro-organisms. An ideal toothpaste to use when there is mouth Candidiasis is Thursday Plantation's tea-tree oil paste, as this essential oil has strong anti-fungal properties.

THROAT INFECTION

A chronically infected throat, whether it involves tonsillitis or not, can lead to a foul breath due to the septic debris in the area. If a throat infection is due to Candida then the treatment is as described above. If it is due to allergy or sensitivity problems then the approach is the same as for other mouth and tongue problems – see pages 49–52.

More typically, however, such conditions are due to viral or bacterial infection taking advantage of the toxic state in these filter (lymphatic) tissues, with allergy sometimes a cause of this and Candida an accompanying complication. Over the years, if the condition is chronic, the tissues of the tonsils can become scarred, making them less easy to heal.

Once a diagnosis has been established – and a qualified health-care professional such as a naturopath or homoeopath needs to do this so that the various causes can be properly assessed – then a nutritional approach for getting the area back to normal is best. If antibiotics have been used many times in the past this will be less easy to accomplish, but far from impossible.

Supplements for Tonsillitis

Local ease of throat irritation can be gained by gargling with warm, lightly salted water several times a day. Other supplementary help includes:

- Echinacea C tablets – chewed three or four times daily between meals.
- EHB (echinacea, hydrastis and berberis) tablets – twice daily with food. These herbs deal with bacterial and viral organisms without side effects.
- Vitamin C – 5 grams a day in divided doses until the condition normalises.
- Vitamin A – 10,000IU daily to help heal damaged tissue, taken throughout the day.
- Zinc gluconate lozenges – sucked several times daily to reduce viral activity and to promote tissue healing.

- A high potency multimineral/multivitamin capsule.

Fasting: A Gentle Detoxification Approach

Fasting is an amazing, proven way of harnessing the self-restorative and healing capacity of the body. Fasting produces two major benefits. The first is a speeding up of elimination of toxic wastes in the tissues – this is known as detoxification. The second is a marked boost to immune defence function, allowing a more rapid control of infection.

If infection or general toxicity is the cause of a health problem a series of short fasts is the best method for restoration of health, especially if the problem is accompanied by constant intermittent fever. Under controlled conditions, where there is expert supervision, fasting can be safely allowed to continue for some weeks; but in the home, without supervision, short fasts only are recommended. The increased immune efficiency is in fact more noticeable during the first 36 hours of a fast, which suits home fasting perfectly. Short fasts are perfectly safe if you follow the simple instructions given below and should be used for any infection, anywhere in the body – not just for tonsillitis.

Before deciding to fast take advice from a health professional to help you select the degree of intensity with which you should apply the various methods available. Choices include water only, juice only, fruit only, one food only, and so on. If you are robust and vital a more vigorous program will be needed than if you are unwell and somewhat fragile in your health. Are you well enough to undertake rapid and active detoxification or is it better to string the process out in order to do the job slowly? You may need to consult a naturopath, skilled in the use of fasting, for advice on this.

NOTE

The methods listed in the series of short modified fasts are safe for almost everyone, but do check with your health adviser first. IF YOU ARE A RECOVERING DRUG USER OR ALCOHOLIC OR HAVE AN EATING DISORDER OR ARE A DIABETIC THEN DO NOT APPLY THESE METHODS WITHOUT ASKING FOR COMPETENT PROFESSIONAL ADVICE FIRST.

The Home Fasting Programme

Over *almost every* weekend for a few months (and thereafter once a month at least for not less than a year) choose between:

WATER-ONLY FAST

This can be from 24 to 36 hours, or if you are fit and vital it can last 48 hours, conducted over a weekend: all day Saturday starting Friday evening and ending Saturday evening (24 hours), or Friday night to Sunday morning (36 hours) or evening (48 hours), so that work schedules are not interfered with. Make sure that not less than four and not more than eight pints of water are consumed during the day.

On the Sunday (if you stop the fast on the Saturday night or on the Sunday morning) have a first meal of lightly stewed pears or apples, (no sugar), or a few spoonsful of yogurt, or a little plain vegetable stew or soup. For the rest of the day have raw food only (fruit or salad), or lightly stewed or steamed vegetables only, or stewed fruit (if digestion is sensitive) very well chewed. Drink as much water as you want, but not less than three pints.

JUICE-ONLY FAST

Have a glass of warm water on waking containing the juice of half a lemon. During the day drink pure water plus at least two pints of a mixture of carrot and celery juice (eight ounces of actual juice each) or carrot and spinach and cucumber (eight ounces/four ounces/four ounces). These juices are recommended by leading American naturopaths for bad breath problems involving tonsillitis, as well as for mouth problems of various types.

FULL WEEKEND MONODIET

Start on Friday night and go through to Sunday evening on a single food. You can eat up to three pounds daily of any single fruit such as grapes, apples, pears (best choice if an allergy history exists) or papaya (ideal if digestive problems exist). Alternatively eat only brown rice or buckwheat or millet or potatoes (skin and all) – boiled and eaten whenever desired. You can have up to a pound dry weight of any of the grains (made palatable by the addition of a little lemon juice and olive oil) or three pounds of potatoes daily.

Whichever type of weekend mini-fast you choose make sure you rest and keep warm and have no engagements – this is a time to allow all available energy to focus on the repairing and cleansing processes of detoxification. If constipation occurs during the fast do not worry – it will normalise afterwards. If constipation is a chronic problem, see chapter 11, which deals with that subject.

In between these weekend detoxification intensives, a milder mid-week programme of detoxification should involve the following pattern (unless any items are known to cause sensitivity or allergy reactions):

BREAKFAST

Fresh fruit (raw or lightly cooked – no sweetening) and live low-fat yogurt
or
Home-made muesli (seeds and nuts and grains) and live low-fat yogurt
or
Cooked grains (buckwheat, millet, linseed, barley, rice, etc.) and live low-fat yogurt

Leave out the yogurt for the first few weeks of the tonsillitis treatment unless Candida is also a problem or unless antibiotics have been used recently.

Drink herbal tea (linden blossom, chamomile, mint, sage, lemon verbena) or lemon and hot water with no sweetening.

LUNCH AND SUPPER

One of these should be a raw salad with jacket potato or brown rice and either bean curd (tofu) or low-fat cheese or nuts and seeds. Or, if raw food is a problem, a stir-fried vegetable and tofu meal *or* steamed vegetables *or* home-made vegetable soup, eaten with potato or rice together with low-fat cheese or nuts and seeds. Chew well!

The other main meal should be either fish, chicken, game or a vegetarian savoury (a pulse and grain combination) and vegetables lightly steamed, baked or stir-fried. Avoid strong spices and go easy on salt.

For desserts have lightly stewed fruit (add apple or lemon juice, not sugar) or live natural low-fat yogurt.

Season food with garlic and herbs, avoiding salt as much as possible. Eat slowly, chew well, don't drink with meals and consume at least two pints of liquid daily between meals. Take the supplements listed on pp.60–61 for tonsillitis.

In early days (the first few weekends) you could

develop a headache and furred tongue with the fast or monodiet – this is normal. Headaches will slowly get less frequent and intense as detoxification progresses. TAKE NOTHING TO STOP THE HEADACHE, JUST REST AS MUCH AS YOU CAN. As the weeks pass, with repetitive detoxification efforts of this sort, your skin and eyes should become clearer (your skin may get a bit spotty for a while), brain sharper, digestion more efficient, your energy levels should rise and you should regain a feeling of youthful clarity you had forgotten – and your throat and tonsils (and sinuses, if these are a problem too) should get progressively more normal as immune function improves.

When the tongue no longer becomes furred with the weekend detox and headaches no longer appear, you can begin to spread these intensive detoxification/fasting weekends apart – three a month and then two a month and then maintenance of once a month.

There are a variety of ways of helping to enhance the effects of the mini-fasts such as Epsom salts baths, skin-brushing, deep relaxation, adequate rest and light exercise. The recommended reading list at the end of the book will guide you as to sources of information on these important additions to the detoxification process.

Once overall health improvement is well established and the tonsillitis symptoms are improving, the in-between eating pattern can also be relaxed a bit with the inclusion of a few 'naughty but nice' easy toxins from time to time – making your social life more relaxed. At this time the supplementation programme can be reduced to half.

CHAPTER SEVEN

Sinus Problems

Inflammation of the nasal sinuses can produce a very bad odour on the breath, especially the breath leaving the nose, and can result from allergy (dairy produce and hay fever allergies are common precursors of sinus inflammation and congestion) or from infection, sometimes of Candida yeast. When such conditions are chronic they are most likely to have an effect on the breath.

If this is the case then the treatment methods suggested on pages 51–59 for throat and mouth problems relating to allergy and/or Candida should be applied precisely as described. If bacterial infection is involved (and more than half sinus problems do have bacterial involvement), whether this is a recurrent situation or a rare event, acute or chronic, then the application of short fasts will boost immune function and help to speed the normalisation of the problem as explained in the previous chapter. Specific supplementation for the sinus region is described below.

Obviously if smoking is part of the problem this should be stopped completely, and if anyone else is smoking in the home or workplace every effort needs to be made to avoid inhalation of second-hand smoke, even if this means use of a mask.

Among the symptoms of sinus problems are headaches, loss of a sense of smell, facial pain, earache and toothache, as the nerves of the region become hyper-sensitive.

Many people use undue force trying to clear the nose, and this often forces material more deeply into the recesses of the region. It is safer, if noisier and less pleasant, to inhale the mucus and let it go down the back of the palate into the back of the mouth so that it can be expectorated. If you must blow your nose do so one nostril at a time and without undue force.

Apart from nutritional treatments such as the anti-Candida diet and programme, the anti-allergy exclusion or rotation diets, and fasting to deal with infection, there are some practical home-help measures that are safe and effective in easing congestion in the sinuses.

Steam Inhalation – The Home Vaporiser Bath

Steam penetrates and can be used to reach areas unavailable to any other method, on its own or as a carrier of essential oils or herbal essences. It is useful whenever there is a painful tight chest during respiratory infections or conditions, a sore throat, or sinus problems. Steam inhalation should not be used by anyone with cardiac asthma or serious heart conditions, or anyone too frail to cope with the heat of steam.

MATERIALS

A kettle and hot water, a bowl, a sheet, an umbrella, a towel, a roll of newspaper (optional), essential oils such as eucalyptus, cypress, chamomile or pine, or leaves such as mint.

METHOD

Bring the kettle to the boil and place it *in a safe manner* so that you can be seated close by covered by a 'tent' made out of the umbrella and draped sheet which also encloses the steaming kettle. A few drops of essential oil or some aromatic leaves can be placed in the kettle and you can also position the roll of paper over the spout to direct the steam towards your face (this is not essential).

Breathe the steam slowly and deeply, avoiding any scalding of the skin by being too close to the spout and taking care not to upset the kettle. Periodically use a cold damp towel to cool the face and forehead. Thirty minutes of steam inhalation, three times daily helps relieve the congestion of chronic sinusitis.

Alternatively add boiling water and a few drops of an essential oil to a bowl, cover your entire head with a towel and place your face over the steam from the bowl (not too close in case you irritate your skin). Keep your eyes closed. Breathe slowly and deeply for at least 10 minutes.

NOTE

The essential oils listed above should be good quality aromatherapy oils, *not* mixed with a carrier oil as they would be for massage. The pure oils are meant to be added to bathwater or for use as inhalations in the manner just described, or via a nebuliser, which turns them into minute droplets. When used on the skin as a massage oil they should be mixed with a neutral carrier (soy or almond oil, for example).

Inhalations for Blocked Nasal Passages

A traditional method for helping restore health to the mucous membranes of the nose involves breathing in either salt water or beetroot juice. Beetroot is the more effective. If you use salt make the solution very weak, just a quarter of a teaspoon to a tumbler of water.

Have the liquid – at body heat – in a shallow bowl as you stand over the bathroom basin. Sniff a small amount up one nostril and hold it there for half a minute before it comes out of the nose again. If you do inhale it right into the back of the mouth don't swallow it but spit it out. Do this every day until the nasal passages are clear again.

Diet for Sinus Problems

For a few weeks, until the sinuses are back to normal, try and stay on a very light, largely fruit-and-vegetable diet, in which about three quarters of what you eat is raw (salads and fruit). Pay particular attention to reducing salt intake and avoid all dairy products (whether you are allergic to them or not) apart from low-fat live yogurt or cottage cheese.

Herbs for Sinus Problems

Echinacea, hydrastis and berberis are all antibiotic and immune enhancing without side effects (pregnant women should avoid echinacea). The combination herbal product EHB should be taken daily for some weeks until the condition has normalised.

Pollen is useful for people whose sinus problems relate to hay fever. A good Swedish or American product (pollen from Arizona is particularly pure) should be used for some weeks before the hay fever season is due and throughout the 'danger' period.

Two capsules of garlic should be taken with each meal.

Supplements for sinus problems

Vitamin B complex is a useful aid, containing not less than 50 mg of the major B vitamins. If you are also suffering from Candida this should be from a yeast-free source. Take one daily.

If allergy is the background to the problem also take not less than five grams of vitamin C daily, 500 mg of vitamin B5 (pantothenic acid) and 100 mg of B6 (pyridoxine). Vitamins B5 and B6 should be taken at a separate time from the B complex supplement.

Zinc gluconate – a chewable version – should be taken several times daily (up to six a day) to help coat the throat and mouth with this important nutrient which controls viral replication.

Sinus problems are not a common reason for bad breath, although it can be the main reason in some cases. The methods suggested, based on diet and safe home care, can help to normalise this nagging problem.

CHAPTER EIGHT

Mouth Breathing

This common problem leads to snoring as well as bad breath on waking and can be directly related to congestion and obstruction in the nasal passages deriving from sinus or other irritation, inflammation or infection. If this is the case, chapter 7 should be looked to for guidance.

Regular – at least daily – use of nasal washouts with mild salt solution or beetroot juice, as suggested on page 71, can help restore the nasal mucous membrane to good health. Placing a humidifier in the room, especially the rooms in which most time is spent, can help mouth-breathers avoid much of the dryness and irritation of the delicate inner surfaces of the mouth and throat that mouth breathing results in.

Most mouth breathers do so because of nasal obstruction, in which case the reasons for this need to receive attention. But many breathe this way from habit alone and if this is the case close attention to the habit during waking hours is called for, along with an attempt to go to sleep with the mouth closed. This should begin the process of changing back to normal nasal breathing.

Regular (at least three times weekly) active exercise which encourages deep breathing should be undertaken – within the physical limits dictated by current health status – along with a concentrated effort to breathe through the nose during and after this.

CHAPTER NINE

Liver Problems

The liver, along with its vital role in digestion, stores essential elements for the body's economy (such as vitamins) and manufactures vital substances (such as bile, which digests fats for us). It also recycles hormonal excretions and is the main detoxification organ of the body, working with the kidneys, and as such has enormous responsibilities and stresses to face when it is assaulted with undesirable chemicals, foods and beverages, alcohol in particular.

The liver also has to detoxify the body of its normal metabolic waste products, such as ammonia from the digestive tract when protein is eaten, and on top of all this it regulates blood sugar levels by storing excess quantities while ensuring the production and conversion of various chemicals that control sugar in the blood.

Fortunately for us the liver is self-regenerating given the chance, and a regular detoxification effort, such as any of those described in chapter 6, involving short periodic fasts or raw foods or monodiets, are an enormous boost to the normalisation of what is arguably the most important organ in the body.

When the liver malfunctions – for any of a number of reasons ranging from infection to chronic toxic overload – it is not surprising that toxins are retained, nutrients are not supplied, recycling is not effectively performed, bile is not adequately produced and therefore digestion not properly accomplished. Nor should we be surprised if out of this toxic, metabolic and digestive mess bad breath should emerge.

HOW TO HELP A TOXIC LIVER

Priority number one is to give the liver periods of rest, and fasting or any of the other shortened detoxification methods described in chapter 6 will do this. Depending on the severity of the situation these detoxification efforts should be weekly (every weekend for a month or two, for example) or more spaced out. The plain water fast is the most effective of these but also the method most likely at first to give reactions such as lethargy, headaches and an absolutely foul tongue. These reactions lessen as detoxification progresses week by week. The fact is that the more strong the reaction, the more toxic you are and the better you will be for the effort. If a gentler approach is wanted then fruit-only diets, a monodiet or a juice diet will be all be effective, but the process will need to be repeated more often for the same end result as the water-only fast.

Obviously, alongside detoxification should come avoidance of the main stress factors for the liver, which are drugs (unless essential medication), alcohol, tobacco, coffee, tea, meat, fried and fatty foods, salt, processed foods, sugar and chemical-ised (i.e. not organically grown) vegetables.

The best foods for the liver are fresh fruits and vegetables – organically grown – along with pulses, grains (especially rice), seeds and nuts. The only oil used should be extra virgin, first (cold) pressed olive oil. An ideal eating pattern would be a grain and fruit breakfast (muesli) with no-fat yogurt, followed by fruit mid-morning, a salad or lightly cooked vegetable lunch (with jacket potato or rice or bread) and a protein evening meal (fish, game, vegetarian combination, etc.) with steamed or stir-fried vege-tables. Drink pure water or vegetable juices.

Supplements for the Liver

- The amino acids l-glutathione, L-cysteine and L-methionine are all aids to detoxification of the liver. 500 mg of each taken away from meal-times each day are suggested for at least three months during which time the fasting/ cleansing approach described above should also be applied.
- The amino acid L-carnitine helps the liver deal with fats and if there is any difficulty in digesting fats

alongside a toxic liver condition then at least a gram daily of L-carnitine should be supplemented, away from meals and away from other amino acids.

- Coenzyme Q10 is a nutrient that helps liver function and 60 mg daily is suggested for the duration of the liver programme – three months is the probable time for a sluggish, overloaded liver to be brought back to normal function.
- Antioxidant vitamins such as vitamin C (2 to 5 grams daily) and vitamin E (400IU daily) along with the important mineral selenium (200 microgrammes daily) should also be taken, with meals, for at least three months.
- Digestive enzymes, which can assist the task of the liver, should be taken with each meal. A variety of products are readily available from better health stores which contain all the digestive enzymes from plant sources. One or two should be taken with each meal.

Herbs For The Liver

- Milk thistle extract (silymarin). This helps to regenerate liver cells – the liver is one organ that can regenerate efficiently given the chance. Silymarin improves enzyme production and protects liver cells from toxic damage. Take according to instructions on the pack – if it is a liquid extract this will be a dropperful (the dropper comes with bottle) morning and evening.
- Artichoke extracts (made from the leaves) as well as dandelion root extract and 'Swedish bitters' (a herbal combination long used as a digestive aid) are all

useful in helping liver function alongside silymarin.
- Ginger is a marvellous liver aid – as a tea or a capsule or added to vegetables in small quantities (grated or cubed).

NOTE

If there is liver infection many of the items listed above could prove helpful but the condition should be monitored by a qualified health care professional. The liver is too important an organ to neglect if it is infected by viral or bacterial or parasitic organisms.

When there is liver infection research shows that a low-sugar diet helps recovery. In viral hepatitis injections of vitamins B12 and folic acid have been shown to help in many cases, and vitamin C speeds recovery.

The advice given in this chapter relates specifically to an overloaded, toxic liver, which may have been dealing with excess chemicals and alcohol for years or which is simply not as efficient as it might be, with bad breath as one of the end results.

CHAPTER TEN

Digestive Problems

There are several potential causes of indigestion, among them a poor choice of food, incompatible combinations of food, and inadequate chewing. Indigestion is also commonly caused by inadequate production of digestive acids and enzymes by the stomach, the pancreas and the liver. Additionally, there may be reduced efficiency or low levels of normal intestinal flora in the small intestine, where much of the digestion takes place.

Any combination of symptoms in the region is possible, ranging from pain, bloating, belching, heartburn and sour taste to nausea and even vomiting. *All* forms of indigestion can include bad breath. Among the most obvious first steps to normalising such problems are following sensible guidelines to eating – not just what is eaten, although this is vital, but how.

HOW TO EAT WELL

Food needs chewing and we have no teeth in our stomachs. This may seem obvious, but eating too quickly without adequate chewing is an often neglected error. The 'Mayr Cure' method described below can help to re-educate most fast eaters. Each mouthful of food should be reduced to a paste-like consistency before being swallowed. This is less likely to happen if the food itself starts out mushy and soft, or if liquid is consumed while there is food in the mouth. The chewing process ensures that the enzyme ptyalin (found in the saliva) is well mixed with the food so that the digestion of it can begin straight away.

Eating with the mouth open, rather than with lips closed, leads to quicker eating and therefore less chewing, so it should be avoided for digestive as well as social reasons.

THE MODIFIED 'MAYR CURE' FOR INDIGESTION

Re-education of the digestive system seems in many instances to be possible if we follow a diet that demands a greater degree of chewing than is normal. In the Mayr Cure you are asked to chew each mouthful of food between 40 and 50 times, so that whatever is being eaten becomes paste. This regime should be followed for two weeks.

Breakfast should comprise a three-day-old (stale) dry roll or one that has been 'dried' in a warm oven. Take only small bites of these, with no fluid at all. Chewing each mouthful 40 or 50 times stimulates the 'satiety' centre in your brain, which tells you that you have had enough to eat, as well as mixing enzymes with the food.

When each mouthful has become a paste, place one teaspoonful of plain low-fat live yogurt in your mouth with this paste, chew a few more times and then swallow. In this way you will eat approximately a quarter of a tub of live yogurt and a stale roll for breakfast. Drink nothing and eat nothing else.

Not less than half an hour after the roll and yogurt, drink a herbal tea such as fennel, sage, lemon verbena, linden blossom, chamomile or peppermint.

For lunch have a variety of lightly cooked vegetables, either steamed or stir fried, together with fish or lean meat – but before eating this start the meal with another dry roll.

In the evening have a dry roll, yogurt, cooked vegetables and a herbal tea. Start the meal with the dry roll and yogurt, and then eat the vegetables. Have the tea at least half an hour later.

During the day sip pure water only apart from the herbal teas, and during the two weeks of the modified Mayr Cure consume no fruit, no raw vegetables, no fatty food, no alcohol or coffee and absolutely no sugar. The amount of time spent chewing is what determines how successful the programme will be. Many people do it every year as a means of eating re-education, weight loss and for general health.

If your bowels do not move each day take a level teaspoonful of Epsom salts in a cupful of water half an hour before breakfast until regularity is re-established.

FOOD SENSITIVITIES AND ALLERGIES

Food allergies can be a feature of indigestion – most commonly dairy produce (cow's milk is the biggest culprit by far) and wheat – and this should be evaluated by elimination diets and rotation patterns as described in chapter 6.

FOOD COMBINING

Balanced nutrition and sound combinations of compatible food are important factors in achieving good digestion. Some forms of food are best not eaten with others – for example it is well established in the Hay system of eating that carbohydrates (starches) do not digest well when eaten with proteins, so that combinations like fish and chips, or eggs and toast are likely to cause indigestion.

Other poor combinations include vegetables eaten at the same meal as fruit, and sugary food with protein. Some fruits, such as melon, are best eaten alone with no other food or fruit.

DIGESTIVE ACID DEFICIENCY

This is a very common cause of digestive problems and is more likely to be a factor in people with allergies, for example children with asthma are very likely to be deficient in hydrochloric acid. It is more common in people in middle age and older.

There are a number of simple ways of testing yourself to discover whether this is the cause of your own indigestion, as well as having medical tests performed by a suitable health-care professional.

NOTE

If you test with or supplement hydrochloric acid capsules never bite them as the acid will damage the enamel of your teeth and irritate the mucous membrane or your mouth and throat. It will do no harm at all in your stomach when swallowed as per instructions, as this area is protected from acid by special secretions.

If you have gastric ulcers do not supplement or test with hydrochloric acid.

Self test 1

From a health store or pharmacist buy Betaine Hydrochloride capsules (with pepsin). Take one of these with a sip of water at the start of each meal three times a day for week and see what happens to your usual indigestion symptoms. Make no other dietary changes while performing this test. Even if there is little or only a slight improvement increase your intake to two capsules with each meal for another week and evaluate the situation.

If there was absolutely no change after taking two capsules with each meal you probably don't need hydrochloric acid for your indigestion and may well need enzymes instead. If the symptoms really improved when taking hydrochloric acid then continue taking them for a time, but also start taking Swedish bitters, a herbal combination that stimulates your stomach to produce normal levels of acid. Take a dessertspoon of bitters in warm water 30 minutes before breakfast and evening meal.

After a month or so begin to reduce the hydrochloric acid intake while still taking the bitters, to see whether the acid levels are now normal. After another month reduce the bitters and take them only now and then if you feel that your indigestion symptoms are returning.

If after first taking the acid capsules there was an initial improvement but not a complete elimination of the problem, try increasing to three or even four with each meal (with bitters), and thereafter follow the advice given above to reduce intake after a while.

Self test 2

Next time you have indigestion or heartburn drink a tablespoonful of either lemon juice of apple cider vinegar. If the indigestion symptoms improve rapidly then you need hydrochloric acid supplementation and should follow precisely the advice given above for taking it – or you can drink cider vinegar at each meal to help the acid levels. If the symptoms get worse when you take cider vinegar or lemon juice then you probably have an excess of acid and should not take a hydrochloric acid supplement.

DIGESTIVE ENZYMES

Most health stores carry a variety of proteolytic (protein digesting) enzymes as well as enzyme combinations for dealing with all the various food types (fats, carbohydrates, sugars, etc.). Obtain a good plant-derived enzyme combination and take two or three with each meal, as well as the hydrochloric acid if this is indicated by your tests. Almost everyone with indigestion can benefit from a period of digestive enzyme supplementation.

FRIENDLY BACTERIA

Lactobacillus acidophilus is the main bacteria living in the small intestine, and it should be supplemented for a few months if there is a digestive background to bad breath. Natren brand Superdophilus is recommended. This is a powdered, freeze-dried bacterial concentrate which needs to be kept refrigerated and consumed away from mealtimes in tepid water – a quarter to a half teaspoonful of powder twice daily.

In addition, *Lactobacillus bulgaricus* (the yogurt bacteria) should be taken three or four times a week to enhance and improve the health of the other friendly bacteria. Bulgaricus does not live inside humans but passes through in about two to three weeks; however, it has a definite beneficial influence on the bacteria that *do* live in us, such as acidophilus and bifidobacteria, which lives in the large intestine.

HERBS

Apart from Swedish bitters, as described on page 86, a great many herbal approaches exist to help both the symptoms of indigestion and the causes.

- Chamomile, peppermint and ginger are among the best known and all can be taken as teas or capsules to assist in easing the symptoms of digestive distress. A Danish version of peppermint (Obbaekjers) comes in powder, liquid and capsule forms and is highly recommended.

- Charcoal tablets and clay (French green or white fine or superfine clay) both help indigestion symptomatically and the clay promotes detoxification if this is a factor. This is taken stirred (a teaspoonful to a tumbler) in pure water (not tap water) away from mealtimes.
- Aloe vera juice is a useful aid to indigestion problems. It soothes the digestive tract, encouraging normalisation of inflamed tissues. A quarter of a cup of water into which a dessertspoonful of aloe vera juice has been stirred should be taken on an empty stomach morning and evening if there is chronic indigestion.

STRESS REDUCTION

To eat when angry or upset is a sure way of disturbing the digestion of any food eaten. It is important to establish a routine of relaxing before a meal, even if for only a few minutes. If you are really stressed it is better to rest and unwind rather than to eat. Practise a form of deep breathing and relaxation regularly and get enough non-stressful exercise – walking, cycling and dancing are all useful and valuable.

Whichever approach you choose in coping with digestive problems, normalising eating habits is a must. This can of course be done less stringently than the Mayr method – it is a matter of personal choice. The various herbal supplements, as well as the option of supplementation with acid or enzymes, are also a matter of choice. Within the spectrum of choices there should be a method that suits everyone to banish indigestion and to clean the breath.

CHAPTER ELEVEN

Constipation

Sluggish bowel movements are one of the curses of civilised society and the cause of untold misery, with bad breath being somewhere on the list of associated symptoms for many people.

Normal bowel transit time in more 'primitive' and less industrialised societies is anything from 18 to 24 hours (the time it takes for food to be eaten, digested, processed and eliminated), whereas in industrialised societies this rises to anything up to 72 hours before it is considered to be a state of constipation. The truth is that almost everyone in Europe and North America is constipated to some degree since they do not have bowel movements two or three times daily – which should be the norm for anyone who has meals two or three times daily.

For the purposes of our consideration of the subject, constipation refers to a condition in which a person does not easily pass a bowel movement at least once a day. Constipation simply means that the waste material passing through the bowel moves too slowly, leading to a build-up of gas, increased putrefaction of the material and the very real danger of possible absorption of extremely harmful toxic wastes.

There is, with chronic constipation, the strong likelihood of the development of localised varicose veins (haemorrhoids) as well as diverticulosis (balloon-like pockets growing out of the main intestinal tube as a result of the pressure of the retained material). Secondary side-effects of constipation include skin problems, a tendency to headaches, insomnia and, of course, bad breath.

The health risks of chronic constipation go far beyond these sometimes nasty but seldom life-threatening problems, however. For example, recent medical research has shown that women who have fewer than three bowel movements each week have a 400 per cent increased risk of developing serious breast disease when compared with women who have a bowel movement every day. The risk of bowel cancer also increases dramatically with constipation, so the efforts to normalise this vital region's function should be seriously considered and scrupulously applied.

One of the prime reasons for this increased risk of serious disease when there is chronic constipation is the effect it has on the billions of friendly bacteria living in our large and small intestines. Amazingly, an average of five pounds weight of these helpful bacteria live in each of us, and when they are healthy they are particularly active in detoxifying our digestive systems – not because they have your and my interest at heart, but because this is what they do as part of their normal life-cycle in the beautiful trade-off that our mutually beneficial relationship has produced. In return we house them and give them nourishment – our food refuse.

However, if the 'food' they receive is excessively toxic or sugar laden, and fails to move along the tract at a reasonable rate, they can become inactive, damaged and relatively poor at doing the things they are supposed to do. And, very importantly, other nastier, less obliging organisms, such as yeasts and disease-causing bacteria, then become capable of colonising the regions in which the now weak and sluggish friendly bacteria live, leading to a range of other problems. So in considering constipation and its toxic effects, and therefore bad breath, we have to take account of the health of the friendly bacteria: Bifidobacteria in the large intestine (including the colon) and Lactobacillus acidophilus in the small intestine (and mouth and vagina).

The primary reasons for constipation vary considerably from person to person, so there is no universal remedy. The causes range from poor posture, which causes crowding of the internal organs and prevents them from functioning normally, to lack of exercise, hormonal imbalances (pregnancy is a common time for constipation to appear), nervous system dysfunction (stress influences this strongly, use of various medications (iron supplements, for example) and, primarily, a diet that is out of balance and contains high levels of processed food (white flour products, white rice, sugar, etc.) and inadequate levels of fibre. If you want a reminder of why diet is so important go back to chapter 9 and read Boris Chaitow's description of modern diet. This summarises precisely the problems we and our bowels face in modern times.

WHY FIBRE IS IMPORTANT

In the words of the leading researcher into this subject, the late Professor Denis Burkitt, 'Fibre increases stool bulk, holds water, and acts as a substrate for colonic microflora (friendly bacteria) . . . and this decreases transit time, reduces intracolonic pressure and produces a softer stool.' Just how effective fibre is in doing this is illustrated by research that shows that if you add just over half an ounce of fibre to the diet daily (say as bran) the weight of stool passed increases by well over 100 per cent and the transit time is cut nearly in half. Quite simply a diet rich in fibre produces a more rapid transit time – material stays for a shorter period inside us before elimination. There are however, problems associated with overuse of some forms of fibre, especially those derived from grains

– excessive use can produce a lot of gas, can reduce the absorption of nutrients from our food and can sometimes cause irritation of the bowel wall in some people. But far more undesirable is the use of laxatives, which force the bowels to open. Fibre improves bowel action through increasing bulk, or water retention in the stool. This produces the effect of stimulating the natural muscular action of the intestines (peristalsis) and a natural bowel movement should then take place without strain. Laxatives such as senna and various patent medications, on the other hand, irritate the bowel to open it, and this in the long run leads to the bowel becoming dependent on more and more irritation in order to get it to function at all.

WHAT SORT OF FIBRE?

The major sources of fibre in food are vegetables, grains (in the form of wheat bran) and pulses (beans).

The fibre in vegetables is excellent, and less irritating or likely to cause flatulence than bran. A medical study looking at the effects of different vegetable diets showed that the fibre from cabbage, carrots and apples will produce similar effects to that gained from bran but without the negative effects of possible irritation and gas. So a first step to fibre increase is simply to eat more fruit and vegetables.

Seed husks from the plant *Plantago ovata* (psyllium) are widely used to increase the water retention of the stool, and therefore its bulk and the speed or its elimination. Psyllium husks are available from health stores in their natural state – when sold by pharmacists they usually contain sweetening or other chemical additives.

Naturally enough, the use of something that increases the water retention of the stool also calls for an increase in the amount of liquid consumed – surprisingly many cases of constipation are caused simply through lack of adequate water intake. Not less than six pints of liquid should be consumed daily in the form of water or juices. This can be reduced if a lot of fruit and raw vegetables are eaten, as the fluid content of plant foods is very high.

As far as many naturopaths are concerned the best way of increasing fibre intake – apart from eating enough vegetables and fruit – is to increase the use of linseed (flaxseed). Linseed is a marvellous food in itself, containing important essential fatty acids, which we need for good health. It also has the property of absorbing liquid, so producing a bulky, gel-like mass that passes through the intestine and stimulates the action of the bowel. It is the gelatinous quality of the fibre of linseed that makes it so attractive when compared to the fibre of grains, which have a harsher quality.

A PRESCRIPTION FOR BOWEL HEALTH

1 Ensure that you eat a lot of well-chewed, lightly cooked vegetables (stir-fried or steamed for preference) and fruit (paw paw, mango and avocado all contain an excellent form of fibre, as do apples, all the berries and pears). Avoid processed products as much as possible, especially white flour and white rice. Avoid sugar and make sure that you follow the advice on chewing given in chapter 10. Avoid drinking with meals apart from a sip or two if essential.

2 Drink lots of liquid – at least six pints daily of spring water and juices, on waking and between meals.

3 To improve bowel health it is suggested that a dessertspoonful of linseed is taken on its own, always from mealtimes, with a glass of water (see Resources page 101). Put the seeds in your mouth, don't chew, just wash them down, and don't eat for at least a half an hour. If normal bowel movements have not started within a few days then increase the intake of linseed to twice a day, at separate times.

4 These measures will themselves help the friendly bacteria to function more normally. However, for the first six weeks of a programme to improve bowel health it is recommended that twice a day you also take, well away from mealtimes, the following friendly bacteria:

- a quarter teaspoonful of Bifidobacteria, together with
- a quarter teaspoonful of Lactobacillus acidophilus bacteria, while at a separate time of day take
- Lactobacillus bulgaricus – a quarter teaspoonful with water.

Ensure that the bacteria you purchase are produced by a method that avoids centrifuging them when they are separated from the 'soup' (supernatant) in which they are grown. Also ensure that the manufacturer states on the package that a specified number of viable organisms, capable of colonisation, will be present per gram at a specified expiration date. The number of organisms that are needed to be useful should be in the billions per gram rather than millions. It is also important that the product should contain live, freeze-dried organisms and should require refrigeration after opening and that it has been kept cool (ideally refrigerated) since it left the manufacturer.

5 For general bowel detoxification it is also suggested that you take with each meal one capsule of deodorised garlic oil.

6 As mentioned earlier, exercise and stress reduction are important factors in establishing regular bowel movements. Take a walk each day or perform some other regular, pleasant, non-competitive form of exercise. Avoid

tension by practising some form of deep relaxation, ideally combined with breathing exercises. Perhaps join a yoga class or do this at home with the help of a book or video.

7 Never, ever, suppress the urge to go to the toilet. If you feel the urge, excuse yourself – whatever the situation – and go. Also avoid straining to pass a motion. If it does not come easily, wait until it does – if you follow the advice above it won't be long.

COLONIC IRRIGATION AND ENEMAS

These methods of washing out the colon or lower bowel are useful at times but can be overdone – they cause a dependence as well as damage to the intestinal flora if used excessively. For this reason the suggestion is that they be avoided unless prescribed specifically by a health-care professional, and then only after the methods indicated above have been tried for at least six weeks.

A colon irrigation can be extremely helpful in ridding the intestinal tract of ancient impacted debris. However, the final insertion of liquid should carry with it bacterial cultures to help repopulate those that will have been damaged and washed away in the earlier part of the treatment.

FINAL WORD

If bowel function can be restored to normal following the dietary advice given above, breath problems, along with a host of minor ailments, will probably disappear at the same time. By paying attention to the entire digestive tract – from the mouth to the stomach to the colon – breath sweetness can be restored in most people and bad breath banished for good.

Resources

Most good health stores and many pharmacies will stock some of the specialised products listed and recommended in the various chapters of the book, such as vitamins, minerals, digestive enzymes, hydrochloric acid capsules, garlic capsules and so on. Better-stocked pharmacies are likely to have a variety of choices for some of the dental hygiene requirements, such as floss, tape, medicated toothpicks, etc., as well as many nutrients and herbal products. Oral hygiene products that do not contain undesirable substances include the following:

Argiletz and Pierre Cattier Clay products Various French clay dental-health products include pastes and clay-based chewing gums for oral hygiene. Some of the pastes also contain herbal extracts such as sage and lemon. Clay is extremely powerful in detoxification.

Bioforce This Swiss herbal range includes pastes made from rosemary and echinacea (a herbal antibiotic) as well as mouthwashes and mouth-freshening sprays.

Blackmore Herbal and mineral oral-health products from one of Australia's leading natural-health product manufacturers.

Comvita A paste based on propolis and myrrh.

Kingfisher A fennel-based paste.

Logona German peppermint toothpaste, Rosemary and Sage toothpaste and herbal mouthwash concentrate for mouth freshening and sensitive gums.

Nelson's Britain's famous homoeopathic pharmacy now markets a range of toothpastes, both plain (homoeopathic) and containing a number of herbal extracts.

Moor Austrian (Neydharting) extracts from plant products submerged for thousands of years are now available as mouthwashes and toothpastes.

Sarakan Herbal extracts in paste form.

Thursday Plantation Anti-fungal and anti-bacterial tea-tree oil paste from Australia.

Tom's This American manufacturer produces pastes that include natural calcium, propolis and myrrh as well as herbal ingredients such as fennel, spearmint and cinnamon. Many of these products also contain fluoride, about which some experts have expressed health concerns when they are actually consumed.

Vicco Plant and tree-bark pastes based on traditional Indian Ayurvedic formulations.

Weleda Pastes include soda, salt and herbal formulations, with specific products for sensitive teeth and baby teeth using abrasive-free gel, as well as gum-strengthening pastes. Mouthwashes containing herbs for oral hygiene are also available.

Specialised herbal suppliers should be consulted for unprocessed herbs, although most of the herbs listed are widely available from health stores and increasingly from pharmacies. A good brand of linseed is *Linusit* – available from most health stores. Homoeopathic remedies and advice are available direct from Weleda Customer Services (tel. 0602 309319).

Some products are imported and not widely distributed, and these are best obtained from their UK agents. For example, Natren probiotic products ('friendly bacteria') can be obtained from Nutri West, Buxton Road, New Mills, Stockport, Cheshire SK12 3JU (0663-742753). Natren products can also be obtained from many health stores and specialist nutrient suppliers such as the Nutri Centre, 7 Park Crescent, London W1N 3HE (tel 071-436-5122). BioCare products are available from Biocare, 54 Northfield Road, King's Norton, Birmingham B30 1JHM (021-433-3727). The Nutri Centre is also the importer of various US herbal and nutritional products such as Echinacea C and EHB (echinacea, hydrastis and berberis) as recommended in chapters six and seven.

The various clay products such as French clay toothpaste and chewing gum can be obtained from the importers Sunny Clay Products, PO Box 3007, London NW3 2UZ, or from the Nutri Centre, which stocks most of the products mentioned in this book. Bioforce toothpastes and their excellent herbal mouthwash from Switzerland are available from many outlets and from the importers Bioforce UK Ltd, Unit 8, Dukes Road, Troon, Ayrshire KA10 6QR (tel. 0292 316664). Blackmores, the Australian naturopathic manufacturers, also distribute widely but can be contacted directly at Unit 8, Poyle Tech Centre, Willow Road, Poyle, Colnbrook, Bucks SL3 0PD (tel 0753 683815). Logona, the German manufacturer of body and dental care products, supply direct – contact them at Logona Direct, Holly Howe, Westhorpe Road, Finningham, Suffolk IP14 4TW (tel. 0449 780152).

The majority of other recommended toothpastes and mouthwashes are available widely: Weleda, Tom's, Moor, Nelsons, Sarakan and Kingfisher brands are found in many health stores, chemist shops and even supermarkets. Some toothpastes, such as Tea Tree Oil, Propolis or Vicco Ayurvedic toothpastes, might be more difficult to find apart from at specialist stockists such as the Nutri Centre (address as above).

At various points in the text readers are recommended to contact a qualified naturopath, for example in relation to advice regarding fasting. These can be found in the Yellow Pages of the telephone directory, or by consulting an osteopathic graduate of the British College of Naturopathy and Osteopathy or of the College of Osteopaths. Dental advice from a qualified practitioner member of the British Dental Society for Clinical Nutrition can be obtained by contacting that organisation and asking for the name of your nearest dentist/member (tel. 071-486 3127).

Index